21 YOGA EXERCISES FOR LOWER BACK PAIN

Stretching Lower Back Pain
Away with Yoga

Morgan Sutherland

21 Yoga Exercises for Lower Back Pain

Copyright © 2018 Morgan Sutherland, L.M.T.

All rights reserved.

ISBN: 979-8-9864227-6-3

Illustrations: Copyright Morgan Sutherland

Cover image: Shutterstock

CONTENTS

MEDICAL DISCLAIMER

The information provided in this report is not intended to be a substitute for professional medical advice, diagnosis, or treatment. Never disregard or delay seeking professional medical advice, because of something you read in this report. Never rely on information in this report in place of seeking professional medical advice.

Morgan Sutherland is not responsible or liable for any advice, course of treatment, diagnosis, other information, services and/or products that you obtain in this report. You are encouraged to consult with your doctor or healthcare provider with regard to the information contained in this report. After reading this report, you are encouraged to review the information carefully with your professional healthcare provider.

PERSONAL DISCLAIMER

I am not a doctor. The information I provide is based on my personal experiences and research as a licensed massage therapist. Any recommendations I make about posture, exercise, stretching and massage should be discussed between you and your professional healthcare provider to prevent any risk to your health.

INTRODUCTION

If you find yourself sitting or standing for long periods of time, there's a good possibility that you've experienced low back pain at one point or another. If the pain is excruciating, you should always check with your doctor to rule out the possibility of deeper conditions, such as a herniated or bulging disc.

Multiple studies have proven that yoga trumped usual care in a 2011 study published in the _Annals of Internal Medicine_. When researchers followed 300 people with low back pain for more than a year, they found that the half who were randomly assigned to do yoga reported better back function (although similar levels of pain) throughout the course of the study.

A 2017 study from the University of Maryland School of Medicine found that a regular yoga practice was linked to pain relief and improved function and might be worth considering as a form of treatment for people suffering from chronic non-specific low back pain.

Instead of popping pain pills and opting for invasive surgery, practicing yoga is a cost-effective alternative.

Not only is yoga a more comprehensive way to stretch and strengthen the muscles and fascia of the entire body, but it engages all the fascial systems that help to hold everything together, providing stability to the lumbar spine, sacrum, and pelvis.

Practicing the following twenty-one yoga poses can help lengthen your spine, stretch and strengthen your muscles, and return your back to its proper alignment.

WORD OF CAUTION

Yoga is usually considered a restorative practice, especially if you have an injury, because many poses are gentle and easy on the body and focus on stretching and flexibility. However, there are a plethora of poses that can cause injuries or worsen them—especially if you already have back pain issues.

If you have a muscle impingement, or any kind of structural imbalance, be sure to avoid poses that overextend your back, forward bend, or twist your body into a pretzel, as they might put too much strain on your back and injure your spinal discs.

That said, the majority of the poses are fairly gentle and meant to be restorative, and you should feel looser and more limber after completing the full routine. In fact, if done before bedtime, you should enjoy a more restful slumber.

1. Chair Pose

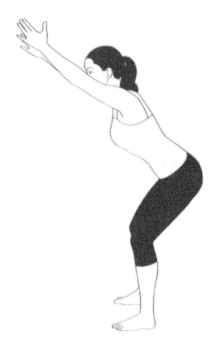

Keep your feet slightly wider than your shoulders, push your hips back, squeeze your glutes, don't lock your knees, and then assume the squat pose. Bring both arms over your head and lengthen through your fingertips.

Pull the shoulders down and relax the neck. You'll keep a lengthening in your back and a tightness in your abs. The weight is in your heels. Hold the position for 5–10 breaths.

How Do You Know When the
Exercises Are Helping?

When the pain moves out of the legs or buttocks and moves toward the center of the low back. Or, if the pain's already in the center, it becomes more of a specific pinpoint, also referred to as centralization. It might become apparent after returning to a standing position. What happens when the pain becomes centralized is that you're pushing the protruding disc jelly back inside the disc, relieving pressure on the nerves.

If the pain continues to radiate down your leg or your leg pain worsens while doing these exercises, don't hesitate to call your healthcare provider.

2. Downward-Facing Dog

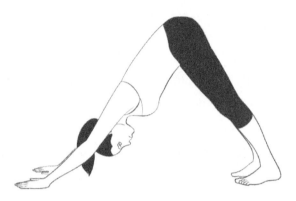

Start on your hands and knees, an all-fours position, with your hands slightly in front of your shoulders.

Pressing back, raise your knees away from the floor and lift your tailbone toward the ceiling. For an added hamstring stretch, gently push your heels toward the floor. Bend your knees, if your hamstrings feel too much stretch.

Hold the position for 5–10 breaths.

What's It Good For?

Besides stretching the hamstrings and calves, the Downward-Facing Dog pose increases flexibility in the upper back and shoulders, while at the same time building upper-body strength.

3. Sphinx Pose

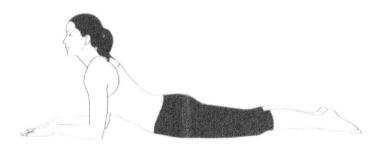

Lie on your stomach on the floor, not on a bed, with legs extended and hands palm down, just above shoulders. Retract your shoulder blades down and in toward the midline of your spine. Maintaining that position, lift your chest off the floor.

Hold the position for 5–10 breaths, keeping the back of the neck long and making sure your front hip bones stay in contact with the floor during the entire movement.

4. Cobra Pose

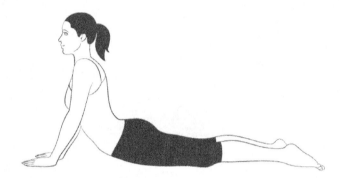

Start by lying flat on the floor with your palms face down near the middle of your ribs.

While drawing your legs together and pressing the tops of your feet into the floor, use the strength of your back, not your hands, to lift your chest off the floor. Leave your legs extended straight.

Hold the position for 5–10 breaths.

What's It Good For?

Similar to Upward-Facing Dog, the Cobra Pose reduces neck and back pain by stretching and opening chronically tight muscles, such as the shoulders, chest, and neck. This pose also stretches the abdominals and reduces the chances of sciatica by increasing flexibility in your lower back, hips, and legs.

5. Upward-Facing Dog

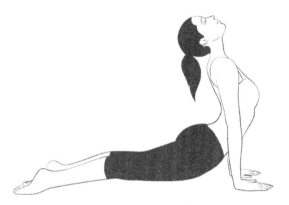

To start, lie face down with your legs straight out. Bend your arms and rest your palms on the floor on either side of your chest. Look straight ahead of you.

Take a deep breath in and shrug your shoulders up to your ears. Squeeze your shoulder blades together.

Now exhale and press your hands down and straighten your arms. Bring your torso and legs off the floor, evenly distributing your weight between your hands and toes.

Try to elongate your body, while keeping your neck long.

Hold the position for 5–10 breaths.

Caution: If you have disc issues, avoid this pose, as it might extend your back too much, potentially compressing the spinal discs.

What's It Good For?

Upward-Facing Dog improves the posture by stretching the chest and shoulders and reversing the desk jockey's notorious anterior pelvic tilt. It also strengthens the spine, arms, and wrists. Another great benefit is that it tightens the glutes, which often get weak from a sedentary lifestyle.

6. Plank Pose

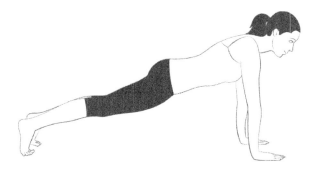

Start with Downward-Facing Dog (see exercise number 2), then move slowly into the Plank pose.

Hold the position for 5–10 breaths.

7. Locust Pose

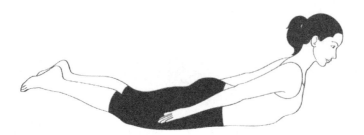

Lie on your stomach on the floor with your arms at your side. Lift your head and chest off the floor. Hold your glutes (buttock muscles) tight, and squeeze your shoulder blades together, Hold the position for 5–10 breaths.

Caution: If you have disc issues, avoid this pose, as it might extend your back too much, potentially compressing the spinal discs.

8. Pigeon Pose

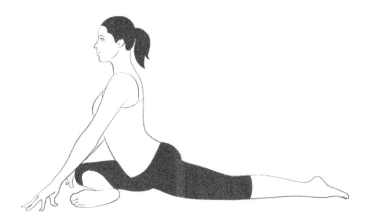

Start in Downward-Facing Dog pose with your feet together. Draw your right knee forward and turn it out to the right, so your right leg is bent, and your left leg is extended straight behind you. Slowly lower both legs. Hold the position for 5–10 breaths, and then switch to the other side.

What's It Good For?

Pigeon Pose can stretch deep into the glutes, releasing the tension in the piriformis, which can cause sciatic pain. The piriformis is a tiny, pear-shaped muscle deep in the glutes that helps laterally rotate the hip. If gets too tight, it can impinge the sciatica nerve that runs through or under it, causing tremendous pain, tingling, and numbness through the glutes and into the lower leg. This condition is called piriformis syndrome.

The groin (adductors) and psoas muscles also get a healthy stretch with the Pigeon Pose.

9. Child's Pose

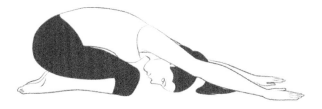

Start with the all-fours position, with your arms stretched out straight in front of you, then sit back so your glutes come to rest just above—but not touching—your heels.

Hold the position for 5–10 breaths.

What's It Good For?

Child's Pose helps to lengthen and stretch the spine, while relieving neck and low back pain. It also gently stretches the hips, thighs, ankles, and the muscles, tendons, and ligaments in the knee.

10. Cat and Cow Pose

Cat Pose

Start on your hands and knees, an all-fours position, and then move into the Cat Pose by slowly pressing your spine up, arching your back.

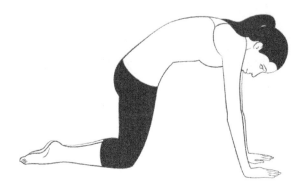

Cow Pose

Hold the pose for a few seconds, and then move to the Cow Pose by scooping your spine in, pressing your shoulder blades back, and lifting your head.

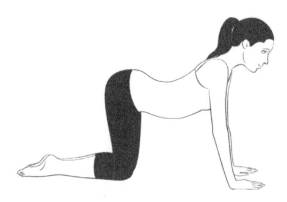

Moving back and forth from Cat Pose to Cow Pose helps move your spine to a neutral position, relaxing the muscles and easing tension.

Repeat the sequence 10 times, flowing smoothly from cat to cow, and cow back to cat.

What's It Good For?

Cat and Cow Pose is great for improving posture and balance. It stretches the hips, abdomen, neck, and back, while simultaneously strengthening the spine and neck.

11. Bird Dog Pose

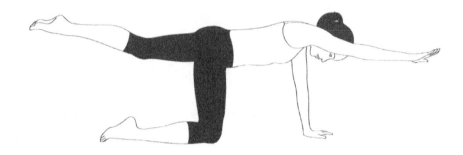

Start with the all-fours position, tighten your hamstrings, glutes, and low back and lift to straighten your leg and opposite arm while maintaining proper alignment.

Hold the position for 5–10 breaths and then repeat on the other side.

What's It Good For?

The Bird Dog Pose is a great core and spinal stabilization exercise, as it helps to reinforce proper spinal alignment and strengthen the core.

12. Low Lunge

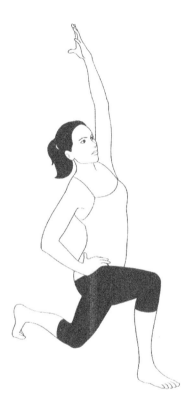

First kneel onto your right knee, with toes down, and place your left foot flat on the floor in front of you.

Place both hands on your left thigh and press your hips forward until you feel a good stretch in the hip flexors.

Reach your hands over your head and arch your body back.

Contract your abdominals and slightly tilt your pelvis back, while keeping your chin parallel to the floor. Hold the position for 10 breaths and then repeat on the opposite side.

What's It Good For?

Due to the predominant, sedentary culture we live in, most people's psoas muscle is chronically tight, pulling on the muscle attachments of the low back. This can cause an imbalance in the pelvis that can ultimately lead to severe back pain or even a herniated disc.

Luckily, by doing this hip flexor stretch, it can help to reverse this phenomenon.

13. Upside-Down Pigeon Pose

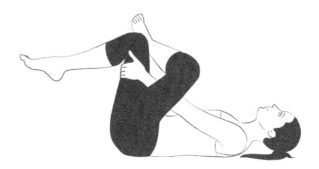

When performing the piriformis stretch in the Upside-Down Pigeon Pose, make sure to contract your abdominals before crossing your leg and resting your foot on the other knee. Hold the position for 10 breaths, and then repeat on the other side.

What's It Good For?

Stretching out the piriformis muscle relieves tightness that can impinge the sciatic nerve.

14. Reclining Cow Face Pose

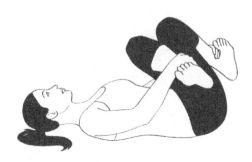

Lie faceup and cross your left leg over your right. Raise both legs off the floor, flex both feet, and reach up for the outer ankles, hugging your legs toward your belly. Spread your toes, keep your feet flexed, and hold the position for 5–10 breaths.

Slowly switch to the other side and repeat.

What's It Good For?

Stretching out the piriformis muscle relieves tightness that can impinge the sciatic nerve.

15. Supine Hamstring Stretch

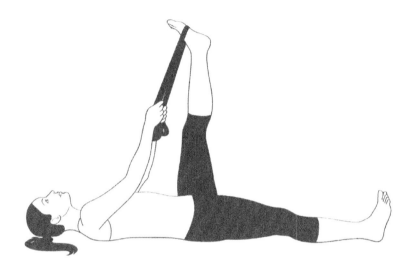

Using a yoga strap or stretch strap has been shown to be extremely effective at increasing the hamstrings' flexibility and restoring range of motion.

Lying on your back, bend your left knee into your chest and place a strap or rolled-up towel around the ball of your foot. Straighten your leg toward the ceiling. Press out through both heels. If the lower back feels strained, bend the right knee, and place the foot on the ground. Hold the position for 10 breaths and then repeat on opposite leg.

What's It Good For?

Increasing the hamstrings' flexibility and restoring range of motion.

16. Spinal Twist

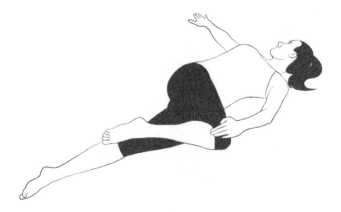

Lie on the floor and stretch both legs out. With your right arm stretched to the right, lift your right knee across your left knee. Contract your abdominals before bringing your knee up and over the leg. Hold the position for 5–10 breaths, and then repeat this move with the other knee.

What's It Good For?

Helps release pressure in the lower back by restoring circulation, increasing flexibility, and correcting posture. It also rejuvenates the spinal column and improves range of motion

17. Bridge Pose

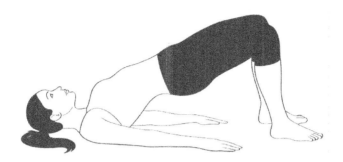

Lie on your back with your hips and knees bent to 90 degrees, with your feet flat on the floor and arms palm down by your sides. Draw in your abdominal muscles and keep them like that throughout the entire exercise.

Hold the position for 5–10 breaths.

What's It Good For?

The Bridge Pose helps to reverse excessive shortening of the hip flexors from prolonged sitting. It helps open and stretch your tight hips, and also helps strengthen the glutes.

18. Happy Baby Pose

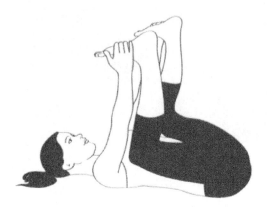

Use your hands to grab the outside edges of your feet. If that's too hard, you can modify and grab your ankles. Pull your knees toward your armpits. Try to keep your feet flat, as if you can walk on the ceiling. Try to keep your chest open and the back of your neck flat on the ground. Also try to keep your tailbone pointed toward the floor.

Once in the proper position, rock side to side, keeping your head on the floor.

Hold the position for 5–10 breaths.

What's It Good For?

This pose helps to externally rotate and stretch the hips, loosen the inner groin muscles, and help realign the spine.

19. Knees to Chest

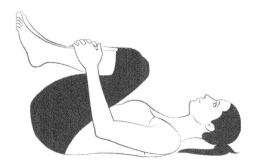

Bring both your knees to your chest. Start by first raising one, and then holding the knee with both hands. Then raise the other knee. Grasping both your knees, pull them toward your chest.

Hold the position for 5–10 breaths.

What's It Good For?

It helps to stretch out the lower back muscles and assists in relieving bloating and constipation.

20. Butterfly Pose

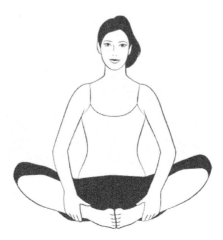

Sit on the floor. Open your hips, flex your knees, and move your feet together. Grasp your ankles and gently pull them up, as you simultaneously push your elbows into your knees.

Hold the position for 5–10 breaths.

What's It Good For?

The butterfly pose is a static stretch that helps to improve the flexibility of your adductors.

21. Legs Up the Wall Pose

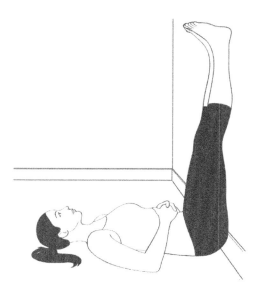

Lie on the floor with both legs extended up a wall. Stay in the Legs Up the Wall Pose for 5–20 minutes. To come out of the pose, gently press the bottoms of your feet into the wall and roll to one side, making sure you support your legs until they reach the ground. Stay on the floor for a few seconds until sitting, to avoid lightheadedness.

What's It Good For?

Legs Up the Wall Pose is a restorative and deeply relaxing pose that brings relief to tired limbs. It also offers serenity and self-awareness to a scattered mind.

REFERENCES

Introduction

Hauser, Annie. "Seven Best Yoga Poses to Soothe Back Pain." See http://www.everydayhealth.com/back-pain-pictures/best-yoga-poses-to-soothe-back-pain.aspx

Wadyka, Sally. (2017). "Try Yoga for Back Pain."
See http://www.consumerreports.org/back-pain/try-yoga-for-back-pain/

"Yoga for Chronic Low Back Pain: A Randomized Trial." (2011).
See http://annals.org/aim/article/1033130/yoga-chronic-low-back-pain-randomized-trial

"Yoga May Have Health Benefits for People with Chronic Non-Specific Lower Back Pain." (2017).
See http://www.cochrane.org/CD010671/BACK_yoga-treatment-chronic-non-specific-low-back-pain

Word of Caution

Newcomer, Laura. (2012). "The Most Common Yoga Injuries and How to Avoid Them." See http://greatist.com/fitness/common-yoga-injuries-prevention-treatment

How Do You Know When the Exercises Are Helping?

"Poses for Your Lower Back."
See http://www.yogajournal.com/poses/anatomy/lower-back

Plank Pose

The Yoga Resource Center. "Plank Pose."
See http://www.a2zyoga.com/yoga-poses/plank-pose.php

Locust Pose

Apt, Marla. (2009). "Learn to Backbend Better: Locust Pose."
See http://www.yogajournal.com/article/beginners/locust-pose/

Reclining Cow Face Pose

Wolk, Victoria. (2014). "Six Simple Moves to Ease Sciatica."
See http://www.prevention.com/fitness/yoga/stretches-sciatic-nerve-pain

Supine Hamstring Stretch

Rader, Julie. "Heal Your Lower Back Pain with These Five Yoga Poses." See https://breakingmuscle.com/learn/heal-your-lower-back-pain-with-these-5-yoga-poses

Legs Up the Wall Pose

"Legs Up the Wall Pose." See https://www.drweil.com/health-wellness/balanced-living/exercise-fitness/legs-up-the-wall-pose/

ABOUT THE AUTHOR

Since becoming a professional massage therapist in 2000, Morgan Sutherland has consistently helped thousands of clients manage their back pain with a combination of deep tissue work, cupping, and stretching. In 2002, he began a career-long tradition of continuing study by being trained in Tuina—the art of Chinese massage—at the world-famous Olympic Training Center in Beijing, China.

As an orthopedic massage therapist, Morgan specializes in treating chronic pain and sports injuries and helping restore proper range of motion. In 2006, Morgan became certified as a medical massage practitioner, giving him the knowledge and ability to work with physicians in a complementary healthcare partnership.

When he's not helping clients manage their back pain, he's writing blog posts about pain relief and self-care, in addition to teaching live and virtual workshops on how to incorporate massage cupping into a bodywork practice. Morgan has received the Angie's List Super Service Award for 2011, 2012, 2013, 2014, and 2015.

Morgan welcomes all comments about your real-life experiences implementing the stretches and exercises contained within this report. Thank you for reading. ☺

Website: http://www.morganmassage.com

Email: <u>morgan@morganmassage.com</u>

OTHER BOOKS BY
MORGAN SUTHERLAND, L.M.T.

The Essential Lower Back Pain Exercise Guide: Treat Low Back Pain at Home in Twenty-One Days or Less

Reverse Bad Posture Exercises: Fix Neck, Back & Shoulder Pain in Just 15 Minutes Per Day

Best Treatment for Sciatica Pain: Relieve Sciatica Symptoms, Piriformis Muscle Pain and SI Joint Pain in Just 15 Minutes Per Day

Resistance Band Workouts for Bad Posture and Back Pain: An Illustrated Resistance Band Exercise Book for Better Posture and Back Pain Relief

DIY Low Back Pain Relief: 9 Ways to Fix Low Back Pain So You Can Feel Like Yourself Again

Printed in Great Britain
by Amazon

38813631R00030